Excel Your Wellness: Virtues and Vitamins

J Pilgrim

Published by Xcel Wellness, 2024.

While every precaution has been taken in the preparation of this book, the publisher assumes no responsibility for errors or omissions, or for damages resulting from the use of the information contained herein.

EXCEL YOUR WELLNESS: VIRTUES AND VITAMINS

First edition. January 2, 2024.

ISBN: 979-8224182756

Written by J Pilgrim.

Also by J Pilgrim

The Trionian Saga
The Trionian Saga - Part One: Beyond the Border Mountains
The Trionian Saga - Part Two: The Hyna Sword
The Trionian Saga - Part Three: The Quest for Lyla
Kass Balou

Standalone
The Hens in Poultsville
Sleeping with Crystal
Excel Your Wellness: Virtues and Vitamins
The Chi Key
Body Strengthening Strategy
Xcel Wellness Tai Chi
The Trionian Saga
Sherleaf
Endless Waterfall

Watch for more at www.thetrioniansaga.weebly.com.

Table of Contents

Excel Your Wellness: Virtues and Vitamins 1

My Early Health Status..5

Step One: Alignment of the Spine..........................9

Step Two: A Naturopath Visit 13

Step Three: A Detoxification Program.................. 19

Step Four: Supplements................................... 27

Step Five: Important Diet Changes 33

Step Six: Relax the Systems............................. 41

Step Seven: Some Amazing Natural Products............. 45

Facts and Tips for Optimum Health 49

Excel Your Wellness: Virtues and Vitamins

<u>Book Bio:</u> No nonsense testimony, wise tips, and advice for the modern person seeking to follow the natural path. Take on the SEVEN-STEP challenge of virtues and vitamins to achieve optimal health and wellness. This health journey has been both a necessity and a desire for the best status for body and mind. It has all worked well. I have the youthful energy and vitality restored as promised by the Naturopath.

Disclaimer: The information contained in this book is intended for educational purposes only and is not a substitute for diagnosis or treatment by a licensed physician.

Unlock Your Wellness Potential with "EXCEL YOUR WELLNESS - VIRTUES AND VITAMINS"!

Are you ready to rewrite your health story? To embrace vitality, clarity, and a zest for life? Look no further! Within these pages lies the road map to your optimal well-being.

This isn't just a book; it's your compass. Let's embark on the SEVEN-STEP challenge together:

Health Status: Rewind to the beginning. Understand where you've been to chart where you're going.

1: Alignment of the Spine: The foundation matters. Align your physical and energetic core.

2: A Naturopath Visit: Seek wisdom from nature's healers. Unearth secrets hidden in herbs and ancient practices.

3: Detoxification Program: Purge the clutter—physically and mentally. Make space for renewal.

4: Supplements: Nature's elixirs await. Boost your vitality with targeted nutrients.

5: Important Diet Changes: Food is medicine. Tailor your plate to nourish body and soul.

6: Relax the Systems: Unwind. Let your body re-calibrate. Find peace in the rhythm of breath.

7: Some Amazing Natural Products: I have chosen to follow the natural path and I would like to present some amazing natural products in this step.

The Healing Symphony.

Clear Mental Clutter: Thoughts matter. Tune your mind to harmony. Let clarity be your anthem.

Balanced Hormones: The cosmic dance within. Balance is the key to vitality.

Purified Body: Detoxify. Shed the old; reveal the radiant you.

Renewed Energy: Ignite your spirit. Feel the fire of life coursing through your veins.

Natural Cycles: Honor the seasons—within and without. Flow like the tides.

Your Empowering Companion.

Facts and Tips: This isn't just theory. It's practical magic. From ancient wisdom to modern science, we have curated the best for you.

The Excel Your Wellness Path Awaits.

Potential Benefits:

Clarity of Thought: Mental fog dissipates. Your mind becomes a crystal-clear pool.

Hormonal Harmony: Balance reigns. Your body sings in tune.

Revitalized Energy: Wake up with purpose. Embrace each day as a gift.

Natural Rhythms: Your body dances to natures beats. Listen closely.

Your Invitation.

Ready to transform? To Excel your Wellness?

EXCEL YOUR WELLNESS - VIRTUES AND VITAMINS awaits. Take this opportunity. Rewrite your story!

The Excel Your Wellness Path's Potential Benefits:

- Clears Mental Clutter improving Thought Processes

- **Relaxes the Musculature and aids Circulation**

- Enhances Inner Harmony and Boosts Confidence

- **Balances the Secretion of Hormones and Purifies the Body**

- Revitalizes with Renewed Energy and Zest for Life

- **Enhances Natural Cycles and Functioning of Bodily Systems**

My Early Health Status

I want to tell you about my health journey. I believe that my journey in the health arena is relevant to many people and therefore highly beneficial. I hold graduate degrees in Thai massage, and Tai Chi. I have extensive knowledge of natural therapies, nutrition, and fitness. I do exercise a gift of observation, and I have a genuine passion for health matters. Any advice given in this publication is genuinely proven to work for many people, but if you are in doubt, check with your health care professional first.

I believe that in any area of life, we must be balanced in our view and propagation of an idea. I do not hold to the extreme of limiting the diet to vegetables, nor do I hold to the extreme of a junk food diet. The middle path is my path, and I hope therefore, to entice you to walk alongside me in the comfortable knowledge that you won't be asked to take too big a leap into unknown territory.

I grew up in the countryside and enjoyed a balanced diet. During my teen years, my schedule was full, and I suffered from symptoms that were physically uncomfortable, but thankfully not disabling. One more point I wish to note here is that when I arose from bed to start the day before 6:30 am, I would be absolutely exhausted by 4:30 pm.

<u>These are the symptoms. See if you have any of these:</u>

- Pressure in the head, headaches, stiff neck

- Fatigue, aching joints

- Dulled concentration

- Sore, tired eyes, dark patches under eyes

- Dull skin tone, dandruff

- Sore tongue/mouth on occasions

These symptoms stayed with me in varying degrees through my teen years and into my twenties and thirties. Being an adult male, I just continued regardless and oblivious to the fact that I should seek medical advice from a practitioner and find a solution to these thorns in my side. In my early adult life, I worked zealously, and I had a kamikaze attitude to my health status. May-be you have the same mind-set today. This is why I am writing this publication – for people like us!

As a young man I could get away with abusing my bodily systems but there comes a time in middle age where this abuse catches up and forces one to investigate the whys and wherefores of health. What we sow in our youth, we shall reap in our middle years. In my early thirties, my status got to the stage where I could not even read a page of a book before my eyes gave way to pain. I was rising up to go to work at five am and come four pm, I was good for bed. I had pressure in the head, tenseness in the shoulders and sore eyes.

<u>My diet mainly consisted of quick and easy meals such as:</u>

- Processed noodles, pasta's, processed meats, processed snacks and drinks

- Frozen meats and vegetables

- Wheat based foods, such as cereals, bread, pasta, biscuits, etc.

- Take-a-ways

- Sugary foods

- Foods which contain Gluten and Soy

I want to note here that I was and am a clean living person, seeking virtues and avoiding many of the prominent vices known in our society, such as alcoholism, narcotics, and smoking nicotine. And yet for all that, I still suffered from these disorders. So, why would that be? The answer is laid out in this publication. I hope that as you read, a light will switch on for you concerning your own experience with similar infirmities. The steps outlined below are remedies that are sure to benefit everyone who adopts the advice given. You may vary within the given framework a little, but it is advised to follow the prescribed path in this publication toward optimum nutrition and health.

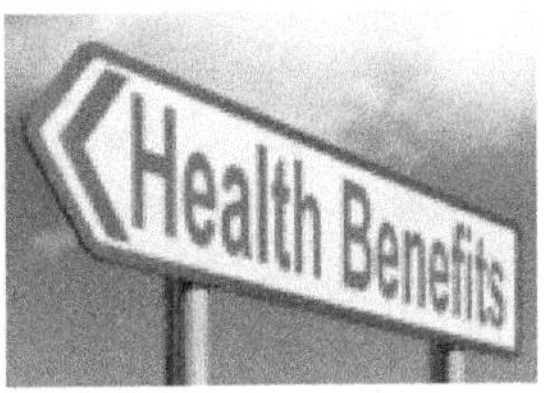

Step One: Alignment of the Spine

During my early thirties, I travelled all over the country in a mobile home. I stayed at campsites and used their facilities to cook, along with other happy campers. It was a go/stop lifestyle. During my travels, I met a man who practised the art of chiropractic manipulation. I told him about my ailments. He convinced me to let him take an X-ray of my back, and we discovered that my vertebrae were out in about three places. There were two vertebrae fused together in my neck region. After a number of chiropractic sessions, I was good to go! The pressure in my head was relieved; my eyes were less bothersome. In the years that followed, I booked myself in for sessions with chiropractors wherever I happened to be in my travels around the country. I learned a lot from chiropractors, just by asking questions and experiencing their different methods of spinal manipulation.

Here is what a visit to a clinic will entail:

- A chiropractor will X-ray your spine to ascertain its condition and curve. A healthy spine will have a slight curve.

- A chiropractor will ask questions about lifestyle and advise on maintaining correct posture.

- A chiropractor will manipulate misplaced vertebrae in the spine back into correct alignment and free up space around the nerves that nestle in the spinal channel.

About fifty percent of the symptoms of discomfort that I mentioned before were caused by nerves being pinched by misaligned vertebrae in various places down my back. I want to inform you that just because you might not feel sharp back pain, it does not mean that your vertebrae are not misaligned in your spinal column. Vertebrae can sit silently misplaced and pinch on nerves for years, causing certain bodily discomforts, and, like me, you just put up with these things because you don't know any better at the time. When people tell me their ailments today, I now know exactly what they are describing. I communicate this part of my story to them, and do you know the usual response that I hear? Some say, 'Oh, the pain will be gone tomorrow. I'll be right as rain in a day or two.' Of course, this response is not acceptable. We must pursue optimal health today.

If misplaced vertebrae are not corrected and remain misaligned for years, then their restricting action on the local nerve group can eventually cause organ failure. Think of it this way – you are watering your garden with a hose and part of the hose becomes crimped: the water flow is restricted. This is what happens to the nerve signals to organs situated in your body. The affected organ (heart, liver, lungs, etc) operates at a diminishing efficiency until it finally gives up the fight. Unfortunately for you and the taxpayer, this usually means an extended stay in a hospital. The sad thing here is that the patient still is not told the truth about why their organ failed. The Western medical system, which is geared towards money-making, will prescribe artificial drugs to combat the symptoms and prop up the failing organ while all the time denying the fact that those long-time misaligned vertebrae caused the misfortune.

In my mid-thirties, I settled down in a town. I booked myself into the local chiropractic clinic, but over time, I eventually became disillusioned with the chiropractic treatment because I was handing over good money for no permanent fix. For instance, my neck would go out within three days of a visit, and I would be uncomfortable again. It was about this time that this same chiropractor recommended I see a physiotherapist, to which I gladly complied, and after a few sessions, I came away disappointed.

It was about this time that I booked myself in with another practitioner to try a therapeutic massage – wow! I knew that I had hit on the best one here. The method of massage is called Thai Massage. The client lies on a mattress on the floor, and the masseur stretches limbs and rubs the body with healing ointments. Pressure points are released with deep tissue massage along the entire length of the back. My masseur began each session by checking the alignment of the hip and then carried out about seven minutes of reflexology before moving up the spine with practiced efficiency. The results are longer-term relief. I continued to go back once a month for a tune-up on my body.

<u>The supremacy of Thai massage is that it:</u>

- Deals with all three – bones, tendons, and muscles

- Re-aligns vertebrae gently and naturally

- Releases pressure points and eases tense tendons

- Rubs muscle fibre with healing ointments to reduce swelling

- Moves lymph through the body to expel it

An alternative to Thai massage is the Western method of massage. This method has the client lying on a specially built table, and it mainly focuses on the back of the body. When you book yourself in to see a masseur, it is recommended that after a few sessions, you ask your practitioner to practice deep tissue massage. Pay attention to the pressure points in the hip region. You will discover that most back problems begin with the hip going out of alignment, and from there, the tension travels up the spine to the cranium, thus producing headaches.

<u>I also made slight changes to my diet and lifestyle at this time, such as:</u>

- New spectacles to help with my eye health

- No coffee - to alleviate headaches from caffeine

- Warm, fresh lemon drink every morning

- Keeping life simple – no massive debt or relationship complications

- Simple stretching exercises

Step Two: A Naturopath Visit

One day, I saw an advertisement in a local newspaper about a Naturopath and the services offered. The headline ran 'Restore Your Youthful Energy.' Tired of my constant beleaguered state, I booked myself in for an hour-long consultation. The practitioner surveyed my diet and lifestyle, made recommendations for change, carried out a physical inspection of my nails and eyes (iridology), and advised me to have a system detoxification. I went away and followed the recommendations religiously for the next twelve months before returning for a review. The practitioner was extremely pleased with the difference that she saw in me and heartily advised me to continue on the same path. I went through another detoxification program at this time too (More about detoxification coming up later).

The detail of what the practitioner first advised me on is this:

- To avoid as much as possible processed and sugary foods

- To eat plenty of fresh vegetables and fruit

- To increase my pure water intake

- To eliminate as much as possible foods containing Gluten and Soy

- To follow a detoxification program

This is the detail of what I did at home:

- I began to purchase fresh vegetables, whereas in the past I had bought frozen vegetables. I used a veggie steamer to cook the vegetables. This seals in the natural goodness and flavour.

- I began to eat more fresh fruit

- I eliminated as much as possible processed foods such as noodle packs, pasta packs, microwavable dinners, and the like, plus sugary foods such as biscuits and cakes.

- I increased my pure water intake by purchasing a benchtop water filter.

- I eliminated as much as possible foods with Soy in them, such as peanuts and peanut butter. Gluten found in wheat-based products was also carefully monitored. In the Western world, this is difficult to do since our staple diet is wheat-based. Nevertheless, rice has become a good alternative.

- I went through a detoxification program. This is a combination of natural nutrients provided either in powder, pill, or liquid form, which, when taken daily for up to fourteen days, will flush stale faeces out of the bowels and harmful toxins out of the kidneys and liver.

<u>The results in the first year were noticeable:</u>

- Pressure in the head, headaches, stiff neck - Reduced

- Fatigue, aching joints - Reduced

- Dulled concentration - Reduced

- Sore, tired eyes, dark patches under eyes - Reduced

- Dull skin tone, dandruff - Reduced

- Sore tongue/mouth on occasions - Reduced

A Naturopath is someone who follows nature's path regarding health matters. A visit to a Naturopath is a vital step to take to excel your health status. Book yourself in to have a consultation, which will generally last an hour. If you have recurring health issues, stubborn weight problems, and regular lethargy, then you may have food intolerance. Food intolerance is a condition where your system cannot tolerate or digest certain foods. The manifestation of intolerance to certain types of food is different for people. Each person must find out for themselves the foods that cause their system to flare up. Symptoms may include white marks on brittle fingernails, irritable bowel syndrome, dark patches under the eyes, acne, dandruff, fatigue, eye sensitivity to light, headaches, and weight gain problems.

Gluten intolerance is more common in the West than people realize. Gluten is a protein in wheat that some bodily systems have difficulty processing. As a result, one can react adversely, giving rise to common ailments. The official name given to this condition is Coeliac Disease. For more information, check out the website of the Coeliac Society.

Beyond food intolerances are food allergies, which are more serious and potentially life-threatening. Food allergies occur when the body's natural defence system sees a particular food in the digestive system as a threat and targets it, creating an immune response:

<u>People can have food allergies to food molecules such as:</u>

- Soy as in peanuts

- Dairy foods - cow's milk and cheese.

- Eggs

- Seafood – shellfish

- Wheat products - gluten

- Red grape juice.

An important step to optimal health is a visit to a Naturopath to determine what your bodily system is intolerant or allergic to in regard to food. By getting on to this early, the Naturopath can detect and prevent many conditions before they worsen to a chronic status. Symptoms are just your body telling you that all is not well beneath the surface. Listen to your body. As you progress on your health journey, you will benefit from a keen sensitivity to your body's internal voice, telling you what foods it does and doesn't like. For instance, when I first went over to fresh vegetables, my body was leaping in anticipation of this new taste sensation. Conversely, when I partook of Fish and Chips one evening, my body let me know that it was not happy with the saturated fat intake. Listen to your body!

In the East, people have had centuries of practice listening to their internal system and knowing that the body is its own best doctor. In the West, we who think ourselves forward are actually backward in this area of expertise. Thank goodness for so many beneficial drugs available in the West, but today, many Western doctors and drug companies are deliberately geared toward throwing artificial drugs at the symptoms of sickness instead of at the root causes. Why? Because money is to be made with repetitive sales of artificial drugs. Artificial drugs shroud the disease for a short season. That's why.

I advise the reader to take note of this and think it through for themselves. Are you throwing away your hard-earned wages on man-made drugs that deal with the symptoms of your illness? If yes, why not rethink your health status today and make a change to follow the natural path toward optimum nutrition and health? Your body is natural: it came from the ground, and it will go back to the dust. Therefore, it makes sense that it craves a natural nutritional solution to prevent and heal itself of disease. It does not make sense to rely solely upon artificial solutions to remedy health complaints.

What is your ailment? Is it a heart condition, blood pressure complications, diabetes, cancer, or asthma? Whatever it is, the immune system is already struggling to rectify the disturbance and requires natural aids in the battle. Instead, we tend to pop pills into a beleaguered immune system, causing adverse side effects. Why side effects? The body may be lacking in natural nutrients, and these artificial drugs may delete certain nutrients from the digestive tract. Artificial medicine can also upset the bodily systems' hormonal balance.

I am not saying that we should completely abandon Western medicine and adopt Eastern medicine, but <u>I am saying that:</u>

- We have to listen to what our body is telling us through the symptoms of dis-ease

- We have to rethink how we are spending our money in our personal health budget

- We have to use sense to realize that our body is a natural organism and therefore will respond better to the natural way

The Naturopath, who will advise on how to follow nature's path, is therefore an important step to take toward optimum nutrition and health.

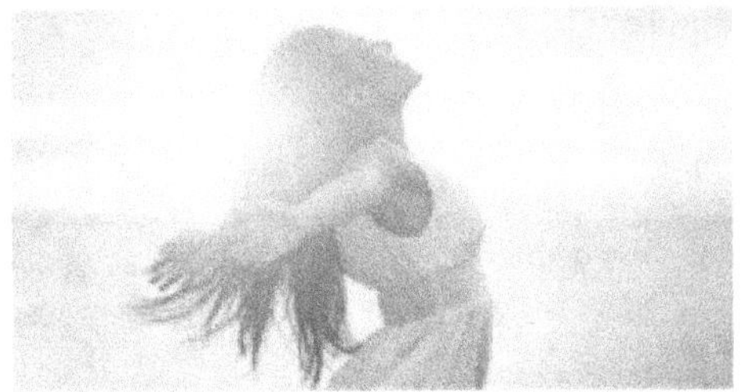

Step Three: A Detoxification Program

As a result of the Naturopath visit, I went through a detoxification program, which I purchased at the health store. This is a combination of natural nutrients provided either in powder, pill, or liquid form, which, when taken daily up to fourteen days, will flush stale feces out of the bowels and harmful toxins out of the kidneys and liver.

The results were noticeable after a few days, such as:

- Being able to think clearly and feel cleaner

- Energy took a rise

- A more positive perspective on life

I researched the matter further and came up with the following:

Detoxification refers to the body's intricate process of neutralizing and eliminating harmful substances.

Several key organs play a vital role in this detox dance:

Liver: The liver is the superstar of detox. The liver, a remarkable organ, diligently neutralizes toxins and aids in maintaining overall health.

Kidneys: These bean-shaped organs filter your blood, removing waste products and excess fluids. They play a crucial role in maintaining fluid balance and excreting toxins through urine.

Lungs: Breathing isn't just about oxygen exchange. Your lungs help expel volatile compounds and waste gases like carbon dioxide.

<u>Skin:</u> Sweating isn't just for workouts—it's a natural detox mechanism. Your skin releases toxins through sweat, keeping you cool and toxin-free.

<u>Intestines:</u> Your gut isn't just for digesting food. It also absorbs nutrients and filters out toxins. A healthy gut lining prevents harmful substances from re-entering circulation.

The digestive system is a significant system underlying a person's health status. Keeping the digestive system clean is crucial to our overall health and vitality. Food digestion in the colon is aided by millions of microscopic, friendly, natural bacteria. There are about eight main strains naturally residing in a healthy gut. These microflora and digestive enzymes are essential to break down and absorb the food that we eat and thereby convert nutrients into substances that trigger essential functions and into energy to power the systems of the body. Enzymes and microflora are abundant in infants' bowels, but as we age, we can lose the right amount and balance of each through over-consuming processed foods, stress, or artificial drug intake. Our natural level of friendly bacteria can take a hit.

The friendly microflora in the colon also works hard to keep unfriendly strains of bacteria at bay. If the balance swings to the unfriendly side, then ill health usually results.

<u>The typical symptoms of unbalance are as follows:</u>

- Uneasy digestion/difficult passage of food

- Headaches

- Fatigue/listlessness

- Aching joints

- Poor skin condition

- Food allergies

- Depression

- Poor memory/concentration

- Acne

<u>Acne on certain areas of the body can suggest a fault in an internal system:</u>

- Acne on the forehead = imbalance in intestinal tract

- Acne on the shoulder = imbalance in intestinal tract

- Acne on the cheeks = imbalance in the lungs/breast area

- Acne on the upper chest and back = imbalance in the lungs/breast area

- Acne around the mouth = imbalance in the sexual/groin area

<u>Feces stools also tell us signs of internal imbalance:</u>

- Sticky stools = liver imbalance. Too much mucus in the system/not enough fiber in the diet.

- Smelly stools = stale food stuck in the colon. Detox is required.

- Undigested food in stool = not chewing properly.

- Light-colored stool = deficient in essential fatty acids.

- Hard pellet stools = Congested liver. Detox required.

- Runny stool = spleen exhausted. Detox required.

<u>Other related conditions:</u>

- Itchy bottom: Worms/parasites in the digestive tract/food allergy/ straining during excretion.

- Difficulty in peeing = imbalance in bladder and kidneys.

- Excessive peeing = Low kidney energy/excessive sugar consumption.

- Dark circles under the eyes = weak kidney performance/food allergy.

- Sore tongue = deficiency of Iron, B6, Niacin and Folic Acid. Poor digestion.

A detoxification program is recommended because it is said that by middle age, there is over a kilo of stale fecal matter stuck in the colon. This lining of the colon walls hinders the efficient absorption of fresh food matter passing through. This matter causes gas, bloating, and sluggishness. In simple words, the system needs to be flushed through.

It is vital to make sure that food moves steadily and regularly through the colon. This is essential for optimal health and the avoidance of many common diseases. The digestive system is also linked to the mind and emotions of a person. If a person is continually stressed and depressed, then the absorption rate will be significantly diminished. Consuming food at haste is not ideal for the digestive system. An eat-and-run lifestyle is detrimental to good health. A mantra to keep life simple is essential for the processing of the food that we eat. Too many people are programmed to think that they have to <u>follow a rigorous path through life:</u>

- Work forty-five plus hours a week.

- have a spouse and children.

- be tied to a mortgage and take out multiple loans and insurances.

- Keep up with the Joneses next door with the latest gadgets.

- Commute on a bus/train to the city center for work.

The above list is there to stimulate the reader to consider their lifestyle and to make changes if necessary. Get back to the natural world in whichever way one can. Feel the breath in nature again. Breathe nature in deeply and learn to relax the systems of the body. Go for a walk on the beach, traverse a gentle hill, or stroll in a bush-clad parkland. Meditate on the positive aspects of one's life, count one's blessings, and take time out.

With the detoxification program, it is recommended to drink about four glasses of pure water a day, and to make this a daily habit. I suggest that one buy a water filter to achieve this purpose. Water consumption prevents dehydration of the body and colon and helps cleanse the kidneys of toxins.

Fiber is essential in the diet to ensure that waste material is moved efficiently through the colon and not left in the system for too long. Most fiber comes into our diet from wheat bran (breads and cereals), fibrous vegetables, and fruits. Water and fiber combined are excellent for the digestive system as they ensure the easy, consistent flow of fecal matter, and they encourage the presence of friendly bacteria in the colon.

A course of Probiotics is recommended after a complete flush of the digestive system. This course involves taking capsules containing strains of friendly bacteria (usually one capsule a day for fourteen days). Actively supplying an abundance of beneficial bacteria helps your intestinal tract to remain healthy. Microflora creates conditions that are favorable for proper absorption. With a healthy balance of bacteria in the gut, one should be free from allergic reactions to common foods, gain energizing blood, and enjoy an efficient immune system. Add to these benefits the fact that these wonderful natural bacteria help the body manufacture vitamins B6, B12, K, Folic Acid, and Biotin, and one can't go wrong.

<u>I completed these two courses (detoxification and probiotics) with amazing results, such as:</u>

- Expelling of stale fecal matter

- Easy and regular passage of fecal matter

- Being able to think clearly and feel cleaner

- Energy/vitality took a rise

- Enhanced immunity

- A more positive perspective on life.

<u>I read up about this subject and discovered these tips:</u>

- Drink liquids twenty minutes before a main meal, not during the meal

- Eat slowly and chew thoroughly

- Take an enzyme supplement to aid proper digestion.

<u>Now, let's debunk some detox myths:</u>

<u>Detox Diets:</u> These often involve laxatives, diuretics, teas, and supplements claiming to rid your body of toxins. But here's the truth: Your body is already a detox powerhouse. It doesn't need fancy diets or pricey products. Instead, focus on supporting your natural detox processes.

<u>Undefined Toxins:</u> Detox diets rarely specify the toxins they target. The term "toxin" can mean pollutants, synthetic chemicals, heavy metals, or processed foods. However, these diets lack evidence for toxin elimination or sustainable weight loss.

<u>While your body detoxifies itself, you can lend a helping hand:</u>

<u>Limit Alcohol:</u> Your liver handles alcohol detox, but excessive drinking harms liver function. Moderation is key.

<u>Hydrate:</u> Water flushes out toxins via urine. Stay hydrated!

<u>Eat Antioxidant-Rich Foods:</u> These protect against toxin-induced damage. Think colorful fruits, veggies, and whole grains.

<u>Sweat It Out:</u> Exercise boosts circulation, aiding toxin removal through sweat.

<u>Sleep Well:</u> Quality sleep supports overall health, including detox processes.

Your body is a detox marvel, equipped with its own superhero squad of organs. So, embrace a balanced lifestyle, nourish your body, and trust in its innate detox abilities.

Step Four: Supplements

Following naturally from caring for the bowel system, I now turn my attention to taking supplements alongside a healthy diet. In my health journey, I have used supplements and found them very beneficial. Supplements are mainly in pill form and are easy to take anytime, anywhere. They can be purchased from any health store or supermarket health aisle. There is a wide variety of nutrients available to prevent and address various health issues. I have found supplements to be powerful agents that strengthen and help heal my previously mentioned ailments. I recommend that the reader try the supplements I have assessed and proven effective, and then, afterwards, experiment with other types.

The supplements that I have tried and proven are as follows:

- Super vitamins and minerals

- Odorless Garlic, Zinc, and Echinacea

- Pro-biotics

- Omega Oils

- Sleep-Ezy (soothing herbs in a tablet).

Generally, supplements supply what may be lacking in a diet with the following:

- Vitamins: A, B, C, D, E, K

- Minerals: Iron, Selenium, Zinc, Iodine, Manganese, Potassium, Calcium, Magnesium, etc.

- Herbs: Echinacea, Chamomile, Valerian, Hops, Garlic, Cascara, Elderflower, Slippery Elm, etc.

With a supplement program, treat the multi-vitamin/mineral supplement as your program's foundation. Build upon this foundation as you diagnose your ailments and add further supplements to boost your defenses and prevent and heal any ailment.

For example:

- If you are lacking in energy, add a Vitamin B complex and also Vitamin C

- If you want improved concentration, add Omega-3

- If you want increased immunity, add a Garlic, Echinacea, and Zinc complex.

The stockist of supplements can also advise on a program that fits your health needs. Most supplements are best taken just after a meal, but some are to be taken on an empty stomach or just before bedtime. The reader can research this matter further.

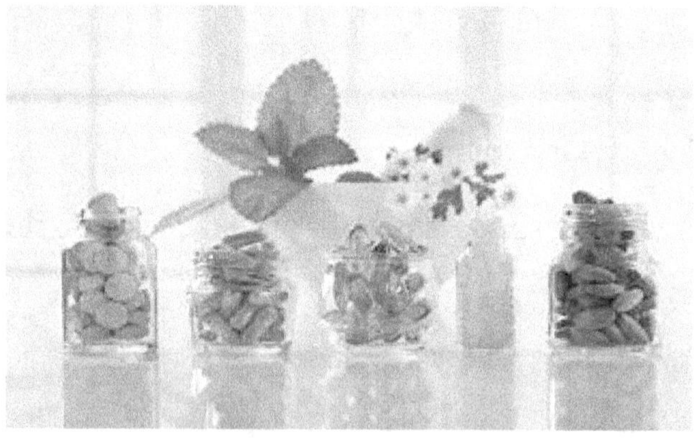

Let's explore the benefits of nutritional supplements and how they can contribute to overall health.

<u>Filling Nutrient Gaps:</u> While a balanced diet should ideally provide all essential nutrients, sometimes our eating habits fall short. Nutritional supplements bridge these gaps, ensuring you get the necessary vitamins, minerals, and other vital compounds.

<u>Targeted Support:</u> Specific supplements address unique needs. For instance:

Vitamin D: Supports bone health and immune function.

Omega-3 Fatty Acids (Fish Oil): Linked to heart health.

Calcium: Slows down bone loss.

Folic Acid: Reduces birth defects during pregnancy.

Antioxidants (Vitamins A, C, E): Protect against cell damage.

<u>Health Conditions and Deficiencies:</u> Certain health conditions (like diabetes or chronic diarrhea) can lead to nutrient deficiencies. Supplements can help replenish what's lacking.

<u>Reducing Disease Risk:</u>

Heart Disease: Omega-3s, CoQ10, and garlic supplements may improve heart health.

Eye Health: Vitamins A, C, and E support vision.

Brain Function: B vitamins maintain brain health and memory.

Reducing Anemia: Iron supplements combat iron deficiency anemia.

<u>Support During Life Stages:</u>

Pregnancy: Folic acid prevents birth defects.

Menopause: Specific formulations cater to women's changing needs.

Aging: Supplements can aid bone health and cognitive function.

While supplements can enhance health, they're no substitute for a wholesome diet. Balance is key—nourish your body with real food, and consider supplements when needed.

Why do we need to take supplements? Don't we get our vitamins and minerals from a healthy diet of purchased vegetables and fruit? The answer if we live in the West is no, not really. The constant use of artificial fertilizers on cropland has, over the decades, depleted most trace elements to a low level in our soils. Any commercial crop grown and harvested could be deficient in many of the trace nutrients that we need. Then, the harvested product is put through a hardy industrial process to convert it into the bottled, canned, or bagged foodstuff that we purchase in the supermarket. Artificial preservatives are sometimes added to manufactured foodstuffs to preserve their shelf life. How much of the goodness do you think is left in the product by the time it comes onto your plate at home? With fresh fruit and vegetables, fresh is best; the fresher the better. If the produce you purchase has sat for a week before you eat it, chances are it has lost a lot of its wholesomeness.

A great deal of supermarket ware is packaged into plastic containers or plastic wrap. Plastic may leach into a moist foodstuff over time. Next time you are in the supermarket, note how much food is packaged in plastic and note how the fresh meat is packaged in the butchery section.

Another reason why people need supplements is when one leads a hectic, stressful, or vice-filled lifestyle with a junk food diet. The bodily system requires extra nutrients to meet the physical and emotional demands.

Some people say that supplements don't work for them. I did try supplements in my twenties, and they did not seem to do much. Today they work well – what's the difference?

I would like to suggest a few reasons:

1: Supplements don't work as well with a diet of fast food, junk food, processed food, and canned food. These terms may portray the typical Western diet today. This kind of diet plugs up the bowels with gunk and, over decades of abuse, creates a picture where one becomes desensitized to what their body is feeling and the signals that are attempting to be sent. Generally speaking, people are in the habit of not listening to their bodies, which tell them what they like to consume and what they do not like. Some people are so 'gunged up' and used to feeling blue that they cannot register any good that supplement pills do for them. Supplements cannot do much good in such a system, as the gunk outweighs the benefits of the supplement. The obvious answer to this is to implement steps two and three.

2: In the above point, we used the term 'gunged up' to express the idea that the body cannot communicate accurate messages because of inefficiency. Now, we address the other side of the coin, which is that such a nutrient-depleted diet is unable to stabilize the health of the bowel system. Supplements pass through the colon too quickly to be sufficiently absorbed. The West has a wheat-based diet. Look around your supermarket and note how many products are wheat-based. It may shock you. A wheat-based diet may be responsible for many health ailments today, with many people being gluten intolerant. Gluten is a protein in wheat that the body finds difficult to process. Over decades, gluten may damage the villi in the colon, and that in turn, causes drowsiness of the mind and body.

I made a switch of diet bases in my health journey. I don't mean to say that we must avoid wheat altogether. That may prove impossible in the West. I do mean that your diet base should be carbohydrates, such as rice and pasta. A high-carbohydrate diet is the ideal diet for supplements to work efficiently. A high-carbohydrate diet of rice and pasta slows the steady movement of food through the bowels, aiding thorough digestion of food and supplements. It is here that supplements work well.

So, with these two discoveries, I now gain the most from supplements and experience their advanced power to aid me in the marathon demands made on me each workday. Supplements cost money, but they deal with the root of the problem, which is a deficiency of active nutrients in the system. Money spent on obtaining optimum health is the family's health insurance in absolute terms and should be the priority. People spend money on artificial drugs that deal with the symptoms quickly enough. My advice is to prioritize natural over artificial and go for optimum nutrition for the benefit of the whole family.

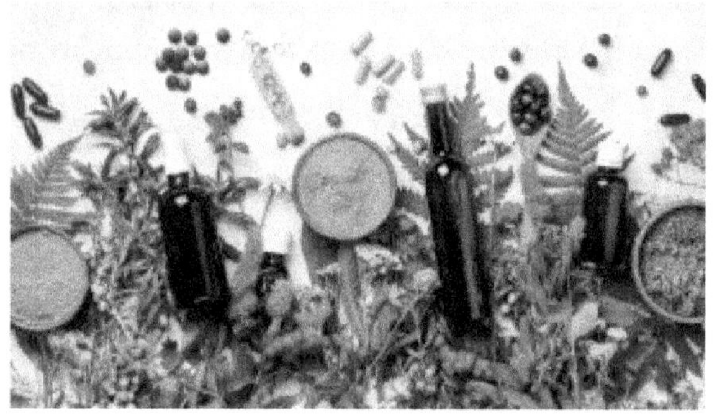

Step Five: Important Diet Changes

Building on the topic of carbohydrates, I want to add more to the equation for optimal nutrition. I have a fast metabolism. If you are like me, you should switch from a wheat-based diet to a high-carbohydrate diet to function efficiently every day. Since I made the switch, I now wake up ready to go in the morning. I will tell you that when I have toast for supper an hour before bed, my sleep is restless, and I wake up feeling slightly fatigued. When I have a bowl of cooked rice before bed, I wake up feeling energized and well-rested. Moreover, rice gives me a head start for the new workday. I also include carbohydrates on my lunch and dinner plates. The professionals advise that half of the meal plate should be carbohydrates, with the rest consisting of vegetables and meat. For athletic demands, this carbohydrate portion can be increased to two-thirds of the plate. The main idea here is to fuel the body! Fueling the body's cells is key to achieving optimal health. Following this approach will help reduce muscle aches and pains, injuries, tension in the shoulders, headaches, and fatigue.

Some people say that carbohydrates add fat to the body. Well, okay, but it is fat that forms a storage layer accessible to the body when it faces strenuous stress. Some fat is good; not all fat is bad. Fat stored under the skin is natural, acting as insulation against the cold and as a readily available energy supply for endurance. The harmful fat is saturated fat, which mainly comes from a high red meat diet and can, over time, begin to clog the arteries—known as high cholesterol.

I am active in my career. I have always had jobs where I am on my feet. If you have an office job or sit in a vehicle for hours, then monitor your carbohydrate intake accordingly. I have a high metabolism rate, which means that the food I eat is processed and the energy is burned off quickly by the body's natural functions. People with high metabolism must work harder to fuel the bodily system. A bit of fat stored under the skin is beneficial. Everybody needs fuel reserves within reasonable limits.

The main point is that if a person's body has no fat reserves and is consistently lacking in nutrients and energy, it must draw energy from other internal reserves. The systems most at risk are digestion, immunity, and cell renewal. Being in this state long-term is harmful and can lead to organ failure later in life. People who neglect their health in this way tend to age prematurely, with wrinkled skin, dull gray hair, impotence, and memory problems. How common is this in the West today?

Add vices to this situation, and you get a dangerous combination that undermines good health. Every time a vice is indulged in, nutrients are diverted from vital functions, and virtue is depleted from the system. Each cigarette, every beer, and any artificial drug intake causes toxin buildup and depletes essential vitamins. Vices are slow killers. People like to think they are getting away with their favorite vices and that life is easy, but as they reach middle age, they face the consequences of their youth.

It's also clear that those who regularly indulge in vices tend to lose their appetite. Smokers, drug users, and alcoholics often show signs in their appearance—wrinkled skin, dull gray hair, and scalloped lips. A decreased appetite speaks volumes about how these habits impair bodily function.

Thus, the natural way—embracing virtue—is the best path for health, both physically and spiritually. Eliminating vices from one's lifestyle can significantly improve health. The real challenge is overcoming the love of that favorite vice. It's necessary to weaken the safety net of vice before gaining control over it.

We must recognize that vice harms those seeking a wholesome, abundant life.

<u>Each time a person engages in a vice, it:</u>

- Diverts nutrients away from vital functions

- Deletes goodness from the system

- Adds toxins to the system

- Adversely affects our personal confidence

- Affects how we relate to others

- Foils the plans for a productive day

- Soils our conscience.

This should be enough to convince even the hardest of us that vice can ruin one's quality of life. Virtues grant a higher quality of life. Let us therefore seek to soar on the winds of moral excellence. Carbohydrates for the body and virtue for the soul are therefore the target to aim for.

Carbohydrates help the body recover after physical activity by ensuring all systems are well supplied with glucose in the bloodstream. The metabolism stabilizes, providing a steady supply to each cell. This is achieved through a high carbohydrate diet during the main meals of the day and evening. My primary hot meal is at noon. This aligns with the practice of many people worldwide and makes perfect sense when you understand the body's mechanics. The main meal should be at midday to energize the systems for upcoming work, not in the evening when the body naturally begins to winding down for sleep. Professionals suggest grazing throughout the day, like cattle in a paddock. This is the natural way. Eating medium-sized meals at regular intervals provides a more consistent flow of energy and balances the metabolism.

Between meals, you can enjoy healthy snacks whether in cereal bar form or as loose bites. And let's not forget fruit as a healthy snack, which provides vitamins, minerals, and enzymes to the body. It is highly recommended that the reader switch from artificial additive-filled snacks like potato chips and cookies to natural snack options. These healthy alternatives to junk food can be found in the Produce and Bulk food aisles of any local supermarket.

<u>What we find in the West, though, is a travesty in this matter, where people:</u>

- Eat the main heavy meal in the evening

- Partake of sugary, saturated fat, and high salt content foods

- Boil the enzymes out of their vegetables

- Rely heavily upon supermarket produce to supply the right level of vitamins.

Eating a diet high in wheat, sugary foods, and saturated fats causes a fluctuating metabolism. This leads to energy levels that rise and fall throughout the day. The result is fatigue when we need to get going and vitality when we want to sleep. Additionally, many people spend money on artificial drugs to manage symptoms of listlessness and insomnia. We need to be smarter and adopt a natural eating pattern that promotes a steady metabolism, supporting the body's energy needs all day long.

Moving on, I have made other changes to my diet that you might want to consider. The next change I implemented was switching from regular tea to herbal teas of various flavors and blends. I did this mainly to reduce my white sugar intake. Experts agree that white or refined sugar is harmful to your health because it disrupts blood sugar levels. Herbal teas are natural products that contain no artificial sugars or additives. They come in many different herbal combinations. Some say that drinking too much herbal tea, especially green tea, may not be good for you. I usually limit myself to about three cups a day. Herbal teas steep in hot water (no milk or sugar needed) and can give you a little boost. Each herb in the teas stimulates a specific part of your body. Some blends help you relax, while others with Ginseng can help energize you for the workday.

A few years into my health journey, I learned the importance of not consuming beverages during a meal. If you think about it, if one drinks during a meal, then as far as the stomach is concerned, you are living on soup. The digestive tract needs solids and fiber to work at its best – this is not achieved when one drowns their hot meal in liquid refreshment. I drink about twenty or thirty minutes before a meal. This prevents dehydration and allows the liquid to be processed before the solids enter the gut. I noticed a gradual but decisive change in my digestive ailment when I coupled this practice with step three.

Another area where I use herbs is in my cooking. I buy mixed herbs like Rosemary, Sage, Oregano, Thyme, Parsley, and Basil. Rosemary helps with cell renewal and memory. The other herbs taken daily will help fight the onset of free radicals and will lower blood pressure. Using more herbs and spices and less sugar, salt, and fat can help improve the overall health benefits and flavor of the foods that we eat every day. Instead of salt, use common herbs like Oregano, Parsley, or Basil to bring out the natural flavors in a meal. The herb Garlic is classed as a superfood, packed full of goodness for the immune and reproductive systems. Rosemary, Oregano, Thyme, and Basil can help fight colds and flu. All four are potent antioxidants, which means that they help purify the body of toxins. The spices Curcumin (in curry) and Turmeric have anti-inflammatory properties. Ginger can reduce nausea and soothe stomach upsets. Spices like Nutmeg and Cinnamon can replace refined sugar in one's diet.

On the naturopath's advice concerning consuming fresh vegetables, I purchased an electronic steamer that works with a timer to start and end the cooking process. This means that I can walk away and do another chore while the food cooks to perfection, and oh, the taste is just like it has come out of the ground. I sprinkle dried herbs onto my vegetables during the last five minutes of the steaming process. I steam my vegetables as this process locks in the goodness of the food. I strongly suggest that boiling vegetables in a stove-top pot be discontinued immediately and replaced with steaming the vegetables. The steaming times for various vegetables can be found in the instruction booklet that comes with the purchased steamer, <u>but in short:</u>

- Bottom-tier basket: denser vegetables such as Carrots and Pumpkin

- Middle-tier basket: vegetables such as Potatoes, Broccoli, and Cauliflower

- Top-tier basket: leafy vegetables such as Cabbage and Silver beet.

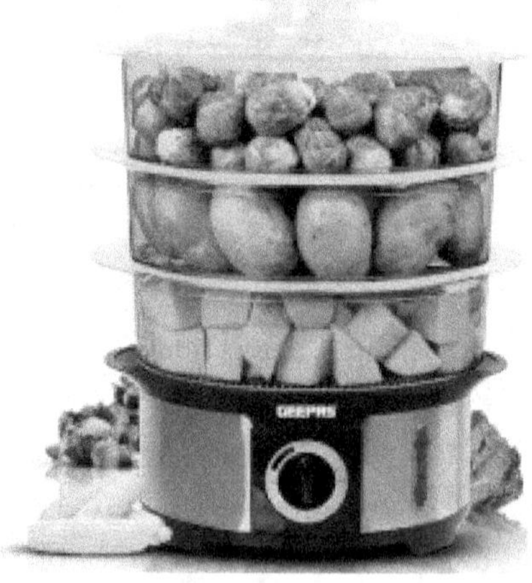

I planted a vegetable garden to aim for fresh produce and planted some of the above-mentioned vegetables. You may like to try to grow your own vegetables as well. As well as the vitamin-packed food you will reap, putting one's fingers in the dirt is the natural way of living. To get back to nature is healthy for the body and soul. Breathe in the fresh air, feel the sunlight on your back, and listen to the birds and bees. This therapeutic exercise is free!

Back in the kitchen, I have reduced my use of the microwave and have instead purchased a Convection Oven to cook my meat. A Convention Oven is a large bowl-shaped device with a rack inside and a lid that contains a heater element and a fan. The small cooker sits on a benchtop and works like a fan oven. This small device is superior to the wall oven as its small size means less warm-up time, quicker cooking time, and less electricity used. It is also so easy to clean.

For rice cooking, I use the electronic steamer, and with white rice, it usually takes thirty minutes to produce wholesome steaming rice ready to go. And it cooks while I am off doing other activities.

One last substantial change that I have made to my diet is around fruit intake. Like many, I was not inclined to partake of much raw fruit. I am not a raw salad/fruit kind of person. I like my food warm and cooked. Still, I knew the importance of fruit intake. I tried an alternative for years, eating some fruit, usually at warmer times of the year, and eating fruit out of a can.

During my health journey, I have purchased a bench-top juicer/blender that processes raw fruit into juice or a smoothie. I add plain or vanilla-flavored yogurt to the fruit mix to make a delicious smoothie. I am careful not to over-blend the mix as I want to preserve the valuable enzymes in the fruit. I need those enzymes to aid my digestion of food. I have my smoothie after I have my morning wash and at least thirty minutes before I eat a meal. The value of this beverage is that it immediately rebuffs the dehydration of the sleeping hours and sets me up for the day to come. I feel good!

I have some Smoothie tips in the last chapter.

Step Six: Relax the Systems

———

Each step in this health journey is a key to achieving optimal health. Each connects with the next, and together they stand. Skipping one step can reduce the overall results. Every step helps calm the body and soul. Relaxing the body is the foundation of good health. Below, I have listed several ways to relax your body and soul. You might also think of additional ways to unwind life.

1: A good, healthy diet. When speaking about this matter, we cannot go past fresh produce and meat, prepared, cooked, and consumed to provide the complete array of nutrients required to fire the chemical actions and fuel the muscles. As we have previously discussed, it is essential to fuel the body so that all systems are charged. A muscle group that is fatigued from lack of fuel means that the tissue holds tension. Tension draws energy away from other vital internal processes, which in turn is detrimental to renewal and well-being.

2: Keep life simple. Going for a daily walk in the garden, park, or shoreline is beneficial. Breathe in that fresh air. Breathe deeply and fill the lungs. Meditate on the present experience and take time out to mull over who you are and where you are in life. Avoid massive debt as much as possible - pay cash as you go. Eschew a mortgage if you are unable to bear its pressure for twenty-five years. Weigh up for yourself whether it is right for you to go into mammoth debt to secure property investment for retirement years or to keep your money freed up so that you can travel, upskill, and enjoy life. Be yourself and take your path through life.

3: Massage and Reflexology. We have already discussed massage in step one. This is a popular method of releasing tension from the muscular system. One can also use Reflexology. Reflexology is where pressure points in the feet are released. The feet contain a map of the body. Each member relates to a part of the body, and tension released in the foot will trigger a release in the related part of the body. Equally beneficial is to invest in a foot bath. To the foot bath, add warm water and Epsom salts. Just sit back and let the bubbles do their good work. If you have a bathtub, fill it up with warm water and Epsom salts and sink back with soothing music.

4: <u>Deep breathing exercises</u>. Deep diaphragm breathing is another way to ease stiffness, invigorate the blood, and increase lung capacity. Choose a form of exercise that appeals to you. I participate in a form of exercise that is soft and gentle, yet effective. The main thing about the exercise that you choose is that it gets your blood moving, tones your body, and engages deep diaphragm breathing.

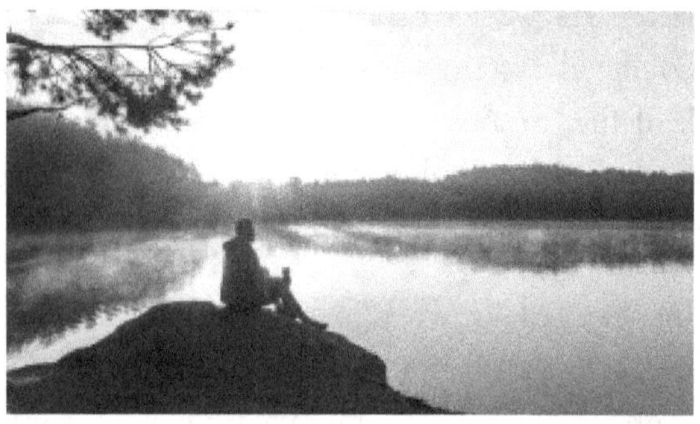

5: <u>Inspiration.</u> From a good exercise program and keeping life simple, you will find that inspiration becomes easier. Inspiration thrives in an environment of ease, where the mind and conscience are clear. You will be able to express your gift most effectively by following my advice in this health journey. I can feel my talent flow when I am relaxed and free from burden and debt. For me, this also means keeping my space from people who will be a liability to me. Choose your associates wisely and join with people who will benefit you in life. People who show respect to my adulthood are welcome in my space. I don't need to put up with those who have angst and create drama. Life is too short for that. My main goal is to protect the simplicity of life, to have a free flow for my inspiration, and to channel my gifts. Your main goal is the same.

Every human being needs to express their special gift and express themselves by following their dream. A blockage in this area of expression is a common reason for built-up frustration in relationships and tension in the body. It is therefore essential that one deals with obstacles and blockages to their expression. This is essential to achieving optimal health. Deep breathing exercises allow inner emotional and physical tension to be released with the out-breath. One can imagine negative energy leaving through the exhale. The result is clearer thinking and a more relaxed approach to the challenges in life. Laughing is also an effective way to expel inner stiffness.

6: Elimination of vices. The elimination of vices from one's life cannot be overstated in its importance in targeting good health. Vices work against the correct functioning of the internal systems and speed up the aging process. The path of virtue is the way to walk if one wants to relax their body and soul. A clear conscience and positive mind are part of the health make-up. To be soft-hearted, forgiving those who offend, and humble enough to confess one's faults is suitable for inner and outer longevity.

7: The seven steps. I would like to repeat that following these seven steps in this health journey will work together to produce amazing results for those who adopt them as a long-term program. The reader has the liberty to move sideways within the framework, but it is advised to stay within the main framework to achieve excellent health.

I would like to suggest three more ideas to relax the bodily systems, which are:

- Natural candles: lighting a scented candle that gives off a natural soothing fragrance for evening close down (such as lavender or sandalwood).

- Herbal tea: choose a flavor combination that relaxes the digestive and bodily systems.

- Herbal sleep aids: a natural supplement that is taken one hour before bedtime and that helps one sleep soundly.

Step Seven: Some Amazing Natural Products

There is a principle in the universe that if one seeks light and acts on the light given, one will receive more light and so on and on, with new discoveries. This is so true of my health journey, as these fascinating insights into wellness have come to me in moments of both action and passivity. I have chosen to follow the natural path, and I would like to present some amazing natural products in this step.

<u>Colostrum</u> is a product on the market that I have tried and proven to be beneficial to my health status. Colostrum, or a mother's birth milk, contains millions of immune antibodies that transfer her built-up immunity to her baby. Cow colostrum is over ten times richer than human colostrum in antibodies that prevent many common illnesses. Colostrum contains growth factors and cell repair qualities. It aids muscle growth and tone. It also contains anti-aging compounds. Users of colostrum report improved skin appearance, bone density, and physical endurance. There are reports of the disappearance of stomach problems, asthma, allergies, impotence, and age spots by regular users. Bodybuilders report that colostrum is an effective muscle-building aid. In summary, Colostrum is excellent in the facets of immunity, growth, and muscle tone.

<u>Colloidal Silver.</u> Silver is a trace element found in the juice of fruits and vegetables. Our body requires silver for a healthy immune system. Colloidal Silver is a natural antibiotic – it kills germs, viruses, bacteria, and fungi. Colloidal Silver can be manufactured and is available from health stores. Colloidal Silver can be taken both internally and externally to prevent and heal many common illnesses. It is an excellent skin healer.

Look at some of the ailments that this product can be used for – <u>it prevents and heals:</u>

Colds and Flu, Infections, Hay Fever, Sore Eyes, Rash, Toothache, mildly infected Ears, Acne, Bad Breath, Allergies, Nappy Rash, Skin Blemishes, Mouth Ulcers, Burns, and much more.

These products are available at your local health store. They deal with the root of the ailment, and there are no side effects. If it comes down to the difference between Western or Eastern, artificial, or natural, dealing with the symptoms or the root, then it is an easy decision where best to spend your money.

What's wrong with Western medicine? Western medicine is based on repeat consumerism – dealing with the symptoms to maintain repeat business. There are products that nature has provided that do as good a job without horrible side effects.

There is a vast market for Viagra, sold to Western men who probably don't realize that Colostrum does the job equally well. Add to this Garlic or any high-sulphur foodstuff, and one has a formidable mix.

Dentists charge the earth to do teeth whitening, and toothpaste containing chemicals is sold for profit, when a humble natural solution like Colloidal Silver is helpful in producing white teeth. (and let's not forget baking powder as an enamel cleanser).

I am an advocate for the alternative way, and this is the message that I would like to promote through telling my story.

<u>I recommend speaking to a health store rep concerning the following health products:</u>

- Colostrum: antibodies for immunity and growth

- Colloidal Silver: nature's antibiotic

- Easy Lax: a mild herbal bowel aid

- Probiotics: containing microflora for a healthy digestive tract

- Omega3: for joints, skin, and eye health

- Protecting/healing herbs and minerals to combat cancer

- Super vitamins/minerals.

My health journey has been both a necessity and a desire for optimal physical and mental health. It has all worked well. I have the youthful energy and vitality restored as promised by the Naturopath. Below are the original symptoms of discomfort, and they are all reduced and resolved.

The results today are noticeable:

- Pressure in the head, headaches, stiff neck – Resolved

- Fatigue, aching joints - Resolved

- Dulled concentration - Resolved

- Sore, tired eyes, dark patches under eyes - Resolved

- Dull skin tone, dandruff - Resolved

Facts and Tips for Optimum Health

I would like to encourage the reader to do further research into this vital topic of optimum nutrition to be well-informed. Knowledge is power - the power to change one's life and destiny. There are plenty of books and websites that give information about this vast subject.

I would like to give a brief summary of my daily program of nutrient intake and good practice. The reader may adjust the program to fit their schedule.

- Rise from bed and wash

- Fruit Smoothie

- Colostrum tablets and Vitamin C supplement

- Muesli breakfast

- I drink filtered water and partake of light health snacks between meals if a bit peckish.

- Lunch is hot with carbohydrates, fresh vegetables, and meat.

- 1x capsule of Vitamin/Mineral supplement

- Dinner is a lighter hot meal with carbohydrates, vegetables, and meat.

- Supper – small bowl of rice

- Sleep supplement one hour before retiring to bed

<u>Here are three refreshing and healthy smoothie recipes that feature fresh fruit:</u>

<u>1: Banana-based smoothie</u>

<u>Ingredients:</u>

1x Banana, chopped

1x Kiwi Fruit pulp

1x Pear, peeled and diced

1x Lemon, juice only

½ an Avocado pulp

1/3 of a 1kg Yoghurt tub

<u>Instructions:</u> Blend and pour into a large mug, add a little boiled water to heat the drink just a tad, stir, and consume.

One can use the imagination and your local seasonal fruits to create drinks that also include:

1x Apple, peeled and diced

10x Blueberries

1x Mandarin, peeled and pips removed

Berries.

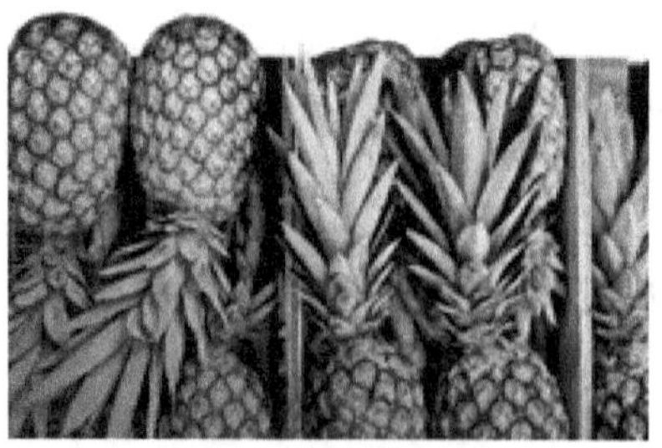

<u>2: Pineapple Green Smoothie:</u>

Ingredients:

Ripe bananas

Greek yogurt

Spinach

Pineapple

Chia seeds (for healthy omega-3 fats, fiber, and protein)

Instructions:

Combine ripe bananas, Greek yogurt, spinach, and pineapple in a blender.

Add chia seeds for an extra nutritional boost.

Blend until smooth.

Enjoy this creamy and nutritious green smoothie!

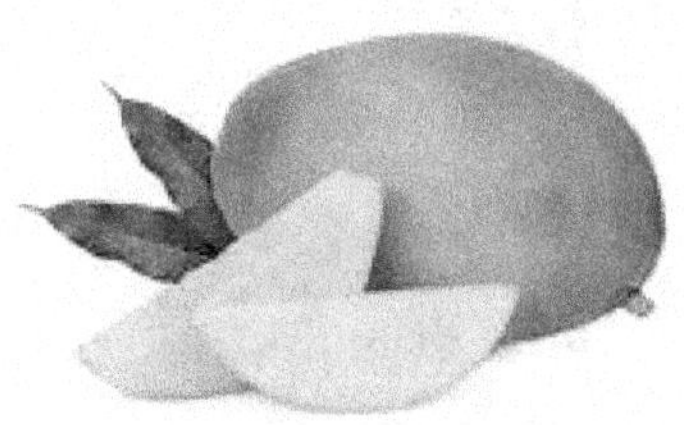

3: Mango Raspberry Smoothie:

Ingredients:

Mango (frozen or fresh)

Raspberries (frozen or fresh)

Squeeze of lemon juice

Agave (optional, for sweetness)

<u>Instructions:</u>

In a blender, combine mango and raspberries.

Add a squeeze of lemon juice for bright flavor.

If needed, sweeten with a touch of agave.

Blend until smooth and enjoy the tropical goodness!

Feel free to customize these recipes by adding your favorite fruits or adjusting the sweetness level. Cheers to a delicious and nutritious start!

<u>I was given this recipe for a fresh lemon drink to combat the flu:</u>

1x lemon with skin on, chop into slices, and put into a pot

Add 1x stick of cinnamon and 1x crushed garlic clove.

Simmer for 10 minutes, strain into a cup, and add honey to drink.

So, that is my health journey thus far, with many more discoveries to make in the years to come, I am sure.

May you follow the path of Vitamins for the body and Virtues for the soul and find the optimum rainbow's pot of gold.

Below, I have listed some **facts and tips for optimal nutrition,** which I hope will whet the reader's appetite to research more deeply into this vast topic:

- Wake up with the sun naturally, eat a hearty breakfast, and engage in deep breathing exercises to ready the body for the day.

- Graze light meals through the day with fresh fruit in between meals.

– Fruit is a fast-releasing sugar to top up the reserves.

- It is best not to eat fruit/dessert immediately after a heavy meal, as the fast-fermenting dessert is held up in the digestive tract by the slower-moving carbohydrates.

- Don't eat late at night before bed or before you are fully awake in the morning.

- Lightly cooked, steamed, and raw foods retain the vitamins and enzymes necessary for the digestion of that food.

- Notice which foods make you feel good and which foods sap your energy away within twenty-four hours of consumption, and take appropriate action to change your diet.

- Eat a varied diet – everything in moderation to prevent the body from developing a food allergy to a chemical in a food type taken in excess.

- Adopt a supplement program and include a number of supplements in that program to prevent and heal your particular ailment.

- Vitamins A and E help clean up free radicals during digestion.

- Saturated fat comes from animal and dairy products. This is the fat that should be monitored in the diet.

- Unsaturated fat comes from plants, nuts, seeds, and fish. This is the healthier fat option for the body to cope with.

- Magnesium, Omega 3, and Vitamins C and E reduce the risk of heart disease.

- Proteins contain twenty-five amino acids, which are the building blocks of the body, necessary for cell activities and muscle growth.

- Protein is commonly found in foods like eggs, meat, fish, beans, and cheese.

- Carbohydrates are a slower-release fuel for the body and are found in foods like whole grains, rice, pasta, corn, vegetables, and fruit.

- Fiber is necessary for the health of the digestive tract and is commonly found in foods like fruit, vegetables, beans, seeds, cereals, and grains.

- Vitamins C and B help turn food into energy for the brain and body. They activate enzymes to release fuel for cells.

- Minerals are necessary for nerve and muscle activity. They are essential for healthy brain and organ function.

- Vitamins A, C, and E are antioxidants and help purify the blood and the body's cells.

- Antioxidant-rich foods are foods like grapes, citrus, mustard, corn, peppers, tomatoes, spinach, cabbage, broccoli, garlic, onions, and berries.

- Antioxidant nutrients keep one looking and feeling younger longer. In other words, they are anti-aging nutrients.

- Free radicals in abundance in a malnourished system can be the reason for premature aging, organ failure, and cancer.

- Excess free radicals cause damage to the DNA of cells, triggering the cells' altered behavior = cancer. Antioxidants are the best defense against cancer.

- Deep breathing with exercise improves the immune system's defense against toxins in the body, cleaning out the lymph nodes.

- Immune boosting nutrients are Vitamins C, B6 and B12, Folic Acid and Zinc.

- Nutrients good for bone and joint health are Vitamins C and D, Zinc, Calcium, Phosphorus, Magnesium, and omega-3 oils.

- Nutrients good for skin health are Vitamins A, C, D, and E, Omega oils, and Zinc.

- Nutrients good for the brain are Omega oils/DMAE (fish oil), Glucose, Lecithin, and Pyroglutamate.

- Excess intake of fast-releasing refined sugars creates a state of stress in the body (hyperactivity).

- Reducing or quitting intake of refined sugar, caffeine, and nicotine will improve brain function as free radicals and the state of stress in the body are reduced.

- Excess intake of caffeine, nicotine, and refined sugar adversely affects bone health.

- An ongoing tense muscle status (e.g., between the shoulder blades) consumes vital energy in the body.

- For maximum energy, have pure food and pure thoughts. A natural body can produce natural vital energy.

- An optimal diet has a high intake of vitamins and minerals from natural foods, fiber, Omega oils, alkaline-forming foods, and slow-releasing foods.

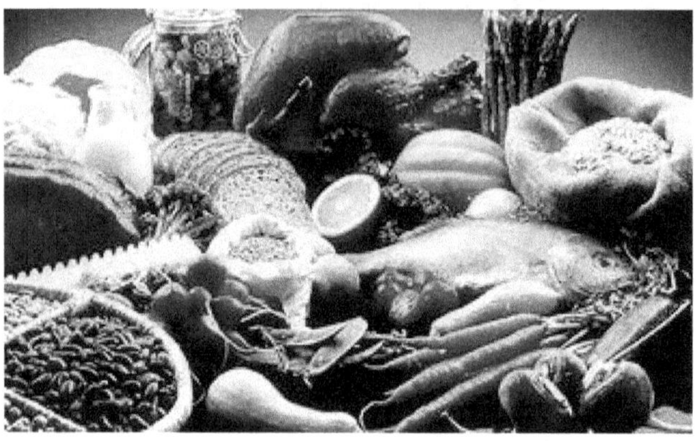

The Power of Nutrient-Rich Eating

Let's summarize the myriad benefits of embracing a healthy diet and how it can significantly impact your overall well-being.

Key dietary recommendations include:

Vegetables, Fruits, and Whole Grains: These provide essential nutrients and fiber.

Lean Proteins: Opt for fish, poultry, beans, and nuts.

Healthy Fats: Choose vegetable oils over saturated fats.

Limit Sodium: Keep your salt intake in check.

High-Fiber Foods: They improve blood cholesterol and reduce heart disease risk.

Potential Results:

Heart Health: A wholesome diet plays a crucial role in maintaining cardiovascular health. By consuming heart-friendly foods, you can reduce the risk of heart disease, high blood pressure, and strokes.

Reduced Cancer Risk: Antioxidant-rich foods protect your cells from damage, potentially lowering the risk of cancer development.

Enhanced Mood: Emerging evidence suggests a link between diet and mood. Nutrient-dense foods positively impact mental well-being.

Gut Health: A healthy gut contributes to overall vitality. Prioritize fiber-rich foods, probiotics, and prebiotics.

Sharper Memory: Certain nutrients, like omega-3 fatty acids, support brain health and memory.

Weight Management: A balanced diet aids in weight loss and maintenance. Focus on portion control and nutrient density.

Diabetes Control: Proper nutrition helps regulate blood sugar levels, crucial for diabetes management.

Strong Bones and Teeth: Calcium, vitamin D, and other nutrients promote bone health.

Better Sleep: Nutrient-rich foods positively impact sleep quality.

Next Generation Health: A healthy diet during pregnancy influences fetal development and sets the stage for lifelong well-being.

Practical Tips for a Healthier Diet:

Variety: Include foods from all major groups—fruits, vegetables, whole grains, lean proteins, and healthy fats.

Limit Processed Foods: Cut down on trans fats, added salt, and sugars.

Hydrate: Water is essential for overall health.

Mindful Eating: Pay attention to hunger cues and eat slowly.

Consult Professionals: Seek guidance from dietitians or healthcare providers.

In summary, a healthful diet isn't just about calories—it's about nourishing your body, preventing diseases, and enhancing your quality of life. So, savor those colorful veggies, embrace whole grains, and let your plate be a canvas of well-being!

So, these are the seven steps of the health journey thus far, with many more discoveries to come, I am sure.

May you follow the path of Vitamins for the body and Virtues for the soul and find the optimum rainbow's pot of gold.

<u>The Excel Your Wellness Path's Potential Benefits:</u>

- Clears Mental Clutter, improving Thought Processes

- Relaxes the Musculature and aids Circulation

- Enhances Inner Harmony and Boosts Confidence

- Balances the Secretion of Hormones and Purifies the Body

- Revitalizes with Renewed Energy and Zest for Life

- Enhances Natural Cycles and Functioning of Bodily Systems

<u>Practice these Positive Affirmations to Re-Train the Mind for Optimal Wellness</u>

- *I Am Vibrant and Alive*

- *I Am Happy and Healthy*

- *I Am Calm and Relaxed*

- *I Am Successful*

- I Am Wealthy and Wise

- I Am Young and Strong

Follow J Pilgrim to obtain copies of his published books on topics such as Wellness, Natural Therapies, and Philosophy.

Involved in the Internal Arts since 2005, J Pilgrim is certified in Thai Massage and is knowledgeable in Reflexology, Gemstones, Numerology, and Nutrition.

J Pilgrim is also a certified instructor in Tai Chi and Easy Fitness programs. As an author, he has books in online bookstores.

www.xcelbooks.weebly.com

Also by J Pilgrim

The Trionian Saga
The Trionian Saga - Part One: Beyond the Border Mountains
The Trionian Saga - Part Two: The Hyna Sword
The Trionian Saga - Part Three: The Quest for Lyla
Kass Balou

Standalone
The Hens in Poultsville
Sleeping with Crystal
Excel Your Wellness: Virtues and Vitamins
The Chi Key
Body Strengthening Strategy
Xcel Wellness Tai Chi
The Trionian Saga
Sherleaf
Endless Waterfall

Watch for more at www.thetrioniansaga.weebly.com.

About the Author

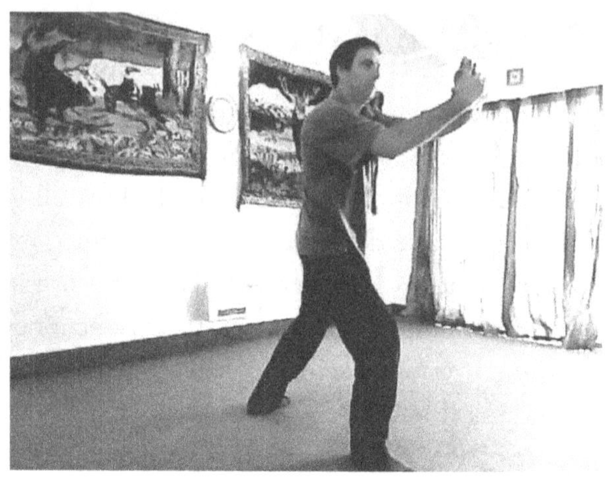

About the Publisher

Xcel Wellness has eBooks published in online bookstores with themes such as wellness, natural therapies, and philosophy.

Involved in the Internal Arts since 2004, the author is certified in Thai Massage, Tai Chi, Fitness programs, and Reflexology.

The author has eBooks published in all good online stores.

Read more at www.xcelbooks.weebly.com.